Breast Cancer at 35

Breast Cancer at 35

---

a memoir

Amy Burns

Fighting Fish Press

Golden, Colorado

Printed and bound in the United States of America by Fighting Fish Press.
First Edition: January 2015

ISBN: 978-0-9906427-5-6

Library of Congress Control Number: 201418028

Cover design by Chaye Gutierrez
Cover photo by Orrin S. Burns

For inquiries, write:

Fighting Fish Press
P.O. Box 7251
Golden, Colorado 80403

Email: breastcancerat35@gmail.com

For the 1 in 7

and for their husbands, parents, sons, daughters,
and friends

TABLE OF CONTENTS

Introduction

It starts with waiting.

I was lucky enough to have found the lump myself on a lazy, Sunday afternoon at the end of February 2012, lying on the duvet with my husband while my one year-old son napped. The lump, if it even *was* a lump, didn't feel *that* weird. My friends asked earnestly, "What did it feel like?" Ironically, no one *talks* about this.

I often wonder, *Why isn't there a touch-and-feel display at the OB-GYN office? Where they'd blindfold you. And you'd hear, No, that's just a rib. Or, yes, that one should be checked out by a professional—see how you can get your fingers around it?* Mine felt like a marble tucked underneath a piece of sliced cheddar on a sandwich. And I wish now that I had just let anyone who asked feel it themselves. Knowledge is power, right?

Ironically, my OB-GYN wasn't concerned about my lump. She told me that on a scale of 1-10, her tiny level of concern was crouching down around level 1. But fortunately, her highest priority was my health and mental security, so she ordered a mammogram and ultrasound. She also knew that my husband and I were entertaining the idea of having a second child, and we agreed that I'd be able to move forward with pregnancy more confidently if we thoroughly ruled out any sign of malignancy. More irony: during the same office visit, I asked her to remove my IUD so we could move forward on getting pregnant again, not believing that the test results would amount to anything.

Two days later, I had an ultrasound and mammogram (my first) and was told to have a biopsy. Another two-day wait. After Friday's biopsy, I waited until the following Wednesday (another five days) for "the phone call." Shockingly, cancer only incites an "emergency mode" as much as the 9-5 business world allows.

Throughout the process of treating my cancer, I managed to continue working full time, missing only one full day of work and a few other partial days for appointments. My surgery was coincidentally scheduled over spring break, and my 9th and 12th grade students in my literature classes didn't know of my diagnosis until later when I was confident that I could tell them everything without breaking down myself.

After my radiation treatments were over and I was on summer vacation, I could finally think. I was ready to start processing. So I wrote everyday while my son napped. And I wrote for *me*, not expecting that anyone else would ever read this...until I showed some of my writing to my husband and to my best friend and to my sister. And they thanked me for capturing what they, too, had experienced. This is their story, too. They are part of me.

But I wondered if anyone else would want to read the story of my cancer. *It's not "bad" enough,* I argued with myself. We are voyeurs for the worst, aren't we? And when it can't seem to get any worse, we still want to hear more. The absurdity of human nature. So at first, I didn't know if I had a story worth telling. Even though I faced trials, my story wasn't as "bad" as others' stories. For instance, I didn't choose to have a mastectomy and opted for a lumpectomy instead, and I was fortunate to forego chemotherapy altogether, despite the doctor's confusion over what to do in my case. My cancer never exited stage 1, and (so far) it hasn't come back. Easy case, right? Not much of a story. Except that it's *so many* of our stories, and this fact, then, is what makes the telling of it legitimate.

I also purposely want to share my story to prove that getting cancer is not always a death sentence—that there is hope in every diagnosis—that not every woman follows the same pattern—that the cement is not yet dry. This probably seems obvious, but I didn't know this at the beginning. I had certain assumptions. Negative ones. Fortunately, my strong faith in God helped me calm my fears and look at my life (which I still had at the moment, anyway) with more clarity. The present was still the present. My response mattered. I was still alive. I was still me. And I had people in my life to love. The second poem in this book is titled "The Decision" based on these precise thoughts. I could fall into anger or I could palpably choose to live. I quickly recognized that it wasn't *what* was happening that was important, but rather, my *response* to what was happening.

The waiting will never end. I'm currently waiting for my next mammogram and hoping I never hear that I have cancer again. But now I wait *differently*. I wait more expectantly. Cancer happened, yes. But this is still my life, and I'm in control of my *response* to the life I have and all it brings.

Appointment

Maybe blunt is best.
The radiologist swivels to face me,
his gray-tweed chair, paltry,
and his office, inconsequential
for delivering any sort of *news.*

"This could be cancer."
His stare follows
like a scratched DVD,
frozen.

I don't have the script.
I say nothing; acquiesce.

Three monitors project three images
like abstract art
like we could sip wine and say of that one,
Look at the lines—
Notice the negative space—
but he's too serious,
his face too dramatic,
and I can't move my lips.
I came alone.
This was just an
appointment.
My keys dangle from my left hand,
my purse
from my shoulder.
I stand in the middle of his sterile office
awkwardly,
like the new kid at school.
Where's the leather high-back?
The mahogany desk?
the "Why-don't-you-sit-down"?
a chair,
or a box of Kleenex?

Something
to thaw the onslaught
of this one-sided discussion—
this moment
like a movie
where he swivels to face me,
his confidence
confusing.

Last weekend,
it was just a lump.
Now,
a biopsy,
and,
I'll pray,
an apology
for my time and anxiety,
a case of being too careful,
a circumvention.

Benign.

The Decision

The March sun of angled afternoons
has turned sideways in its anxiety,
and through our dining room window,
rapes the shadows.
An incoming call,
its vibrating pulse
beating the kitchen counter.

I answer.
Suddenly—our lives
exposed.
Invasive ductal carcinoma.
ER Positive.
PR Positive.
HER 2 Negative.
I'm still listening.

I mouth it to you—the hard C of it choking my
confidence and
catching on my tonsils.
After the news,
I see your eyelids like wet newsprint.
Don't move, I say inside my head.
Everything in this moment is in danger of tearing.
Dissolving.
Disappearing.
But you're standing next to me
on a stone floor
that will not come undone.
And you're holding our thirteen-month-old son
who's reaching for me.
There is nothing else.

Submerged

A deluge of phone calls,
female voices, variation of intonation,
naming
not asking
dates
times
like a conversation
underwater,
their syllables siphoning off
names of doctors,
different floors.

I nod,
realize the voice can't hear my nod,
say, "OK,"
and try to breathe out.
My shoulders and ears are fused to the phone,
my lungs a floodplain,
brackish.

I'm scratching numbers on a Target receipt,
dull pencil from the junk drawer,
hand trembling,
rendering figures hardly decipherable.
Will I remember if that's a 4 or a 9?
I try to fix it—
and make it worse.

I do not have room for this.
My thumb scrolls through my calendar,
feels the new weight of today
and tomorrow
and the day after.

Until the gears halt
right smack at the tear ducts.

They must already know
I cannot micro-manage this.

Digress

My world is clashing with some other.
Like there are too many lights on.
Or the mirror got moved to the other side of the room.
The news...just two hours old.
My hand still squeezes my phone,
my mind, fragile.
I sit on a high pile of shag
leaning heavily against our Craigslist-found crib—
high quality, espresso finish.
It didn't come with teeth marks—
this relic of life,
precious and unrefined.
Next to me, books explode off shelves like 52 pick-up:
Goodnight Moon,
Bedtime for Tad,
Five Little Ladybugs,
Peter Rabbit,
my lap weighted with cardboard adventures;
a small hand touches my knee, asking.

The radio plays softly in the next room.
I instantly recognize the opening chord—
"We are Young" by Fun—
scoop up my son in my arms,
and rush to turn up the volume,
to erase the inflection at the end of this question,
to fix what's been
broken.

With eyes bright despite puffiness,
we dance on the hardwood,
my long, straight hair spinning at 45 degrees
like motorized amusement-park swings—
circling.
Finally, a smile.
From him, too, his head bobbing in my arms.
Then giddy.

My husband, dazed,
looks on from the doorjamb
and sensing a change,
grins.

Playful.
This.

Click below to accept these terms

Here's the paradox:

everything we know about life
stops
at the start
of the unknown.

People speak tritely of how events change them.
Mold them.
Transform them.
But that's only later.
After reflection.
No one talks about
the stopping.
The cessation of time.
The breathing underwater.
The *now* of it.

My husband gently sets plates of leftovers
in front of us
and we tell ourselves to chew.

We have lost the present
because
we are buried in it.
My eyes ensconce my fear,
invite numbness.
No one talks about the stopping,
the hardest part after the waiting.

When really, this is it.
The gritty part.
The real trial.
No head games.
Say it.
Out loud.
I have breast cancer.

The Nurse

After the consultation with the surgeon,
the nurse speaks to me of drains
and Vicodin,
of steri-strips and sports bras,
ice packs and swelling,
and a "good cosmetic result."
Exactitude and obscurity hold hands.
No one *really* knows anything.
No one *really* knows how *my* body
will react
will heal
will cooperate.
So I sit stunned
and nod.
And still, she's talking.

Actually, I do a lot of nodding—
a Hebrew word meaning *to wander*
like Cain, exiled,
wandering in the Land of Nod,
the land east of Eden
like my thoughts
now incoherent
under optical fluorescence—
and like old "to do" lists
and dreams
that I've awoken from
in the middle of the night,
paper by the pillow,
a crosswise script in the dark
and nothing means anything by morning.

The Oncologist

Funny how in that single hour he could say almost
anything:

Your breasts might not match
Your skin might lose its sensitivity
You probably won't have children again
You might have a greater chance of other cancers

But it wasn't until he said it about losing my hair—
a fact I already knew—
was expecting—
the vagaries of my fragile state
uprooted.

Last summer a microburst
induced a sudden and violent
wind shear.
Mature cottonwoods on the I-70 corridor
near my house, defeated—
tendrils of roots suffering in August heat,
gripping clumps of clay
and twitching while the great beasts lay on their sides
like downed elephants.

Look at the place
where their heels dug in—
how the cavernous earth
gapes at its loss—
desperate
to hold tight again.

You're not going to die

is what I want anyone to tell me
but they
and you too
evade even the question
(and God knows) the answer
so we talk about
the plan
because
the plan
is controllable
and clean
sterile
and safe
like your face
facing mine
steady
and faint at the same time
controlled
you will not cry
you will not cry
I know you have told yourself
while shouldering the question mark.

I'm OK
I say
and I really am
have to be
long to be
choose to be
so I tell you that my next
appointment
is next
Friday at 8
the only palpable
hope
something to wait for
to pay for

do
prolong.

That's good
you say
and smile
stretching your lips
waiting to see if I'll stretch mine
so I do
this is a choice
after all
and we feed off each other
I know I have to give you
what you need from me

hope

funny
who's comforting whom?
but it'd be a lot
easier
to say I'm OK
if I knew with certainty
that I really would be.

Birthday Dinner

A few weeks ago I asked you
how you'd like to celebrate.
We didn't know then
that birthday would be
synonymous with surgery.
But they said surgery would take two hours—
it only took one.
They said recovery could take five hours—
it took thirty minutes.
Before they dismissed me, they told me
I'd be out for days—
so I took you out for dinner.
Nobody *really* knows anything.

Holding hands, we walked to Providence Tavern
for the best burger in Denver,
my tape and bandages mostly hidden
under clothing that still made me feel sexy.
The side doors were propped open
on that unusually warm, spring evening,
and on bar stools, we sat proud,
laughing at my condition—
the orange dye I forgot to wipe
from my inner-arm and chest
and the way I protected my left side
when waitresses weaved by.
I sipped your Buffalo Trace with a sheepish grin,
you finished my fries,
and we walked home.

How sacred is normalcy.
How playful is the spirit
when it's unfettered from human suggestion.
How thankful.

Purple

will be the color of my
wig,
I say,
and laugh.
But no,
seriously.
Thank you
for laughing with me,
for camaraderie,
for joining me in
frivolity
like we're choosing flavors of ice-cream
together
and thanks
for the edible fruit bouquet.
I love pineapple.
A gesture.
Thank you, too, for coming over—
for being loud.

Enigma

I am not born of the medical profession.
I do not digest medical lingo by choice
or crave flavors of data.
I am not a connoisseur of statistics
nor wish to add my own
to any website.
I teach high-school students.
I give and expect instructions.

I am standing in the backyard grass
chaperoning the pushing of Tonka trucks
when the doctor calls.
"With aggressive grade-3 cells
but an Oncotype score of 12,
you're an enigma."
I just stand there.
I don't know what to make of this.
I think that's his point, too.
Everything is still up in the air.
Chemotherapy?
Radiation?
Genetic testing?
Further surgery?
I should be glad
I get to choose.
I should take control by its wrists
and yank it sideways.
But I am weak right now
and want simply to be told.

I have to remind myself
that this is human—
the *not*-knowing.
That it's good,
keeps me pushing forward,
praying upward.
That it oddly assuages fear.

This cannot be the end
if it's so obviously the middle.

Enigma, Part Two

"We don't know what caused your cancer."
Another doctor.
Another set of tests.
Another consultation
with hands folded,
knees tight,
and eyes locked.
Such a proper disease.
"...And you *didn't* test positive
for the BRCA 1 or 2 genes."
I exhale.
I was hoping for this.
Though, strangely, it still means nothing.
The family history I had scribbled down
was now color-coded, labeled, and boxed together—
a classification of organisms
a hierarchy of rank
to accompany my blood test.

The doctor hands to me
the four-thousand-dollar test results
earnestly,
fervently,
as if she has helped—
as if cancer behaves better
if handcuffed to a spreadsheet.
We shake hands,
and I leave,
my inconclusive answer
an antonym for security.

Toxic

Noxious, this disease—
"and you're so young!" everyone exclaims.
They need a reason
an answer
an explanation
even more than I.
They want to know that it won't
happen to them.
Like claiming an exemption on their taxes.

I'm only thirty-five.
I'm 5'8" and 127 pounds.
I'm a member of 24-Hour Fitness
and I love kale.
I'll occasionally rush to make happy hour—
press an orange into a Blue Moon—
but I don't *drink*.

Where did this come from?

Maybe, I muse, I shouldn't have
taken birth control,
or eaten food from micro-waved Tupperware,
or stopped going to yoga last October.
Maybe I should have
breast-fed my son *longer*
or stopped cleaning the bathtub with Lysol.
Maybe I should have
eaten more grass-fed beef,
or avoided drinking water straight from the tap.
Maybe it's because my gardening gloves have holes
in the thumbs
or because my Mazda failed its emissions test in '97.
Maybe I forgot to take my multi-vitamin,
or had too much Cheez Whiz as a kid,
or stood in line at the Ogden
next to

someone smoking.

My library books settle in stacks on the kitchen island:
The Breast Cancer Prevention Diet,
The Breast-Cancer Companion,
Secrets from the Sisterhood of Breast Cancer Survivors,
Breast Cancer for Husbands—
their due-date slips hanging from their mouths
like tongues, exhausted.
Each book with a different method,
a disparate set of steps,
an inconsistent menu,
a soap-box solution—
a frustrating contradiction of life's rules.

So I visualize boarding a spacecraft to the moon,
exiting ozone and toxic atmosphere,
and cleaning the core of me
cell by cell

until my flip flops sink too far into lunar dust
and I breathe it in too quickly,
or blink wrong,
or don't get *enough* sun,
and learn, not soon enough,
that perhaps lunar dust is toxic, too.

External Indicators of an Identity Crisis

Inside the tattoo parlor on Colfax
at twenty-three years old,
I waited my turn
with apprehension.
A man with a tarantula
on his shoulder
and large gauges in each lobe
kindly explained the sequence
as I laid on a white table,
belly-up.
A chosen vulnerability.
Two dots with a black Sharpie,
then he cleansed and clamped
my eyebrow tight
threading metal.
"On the count of three."
Then the needle,
the stainless ring
and it was over.
Exhale.

Inside the radiation-oncology wing
at thirty-five,
I wait my turn
with apprehension.
A man wearing a white lab coat
kindly explains the sequence
as I lay on a white table,
belly-up.
Breasts exposed.
The table whirs,
he repositions me—
then disappears to read the ghost pictures
of my chest.
Satisfied,
he draws on me with a black Sharpie—
a full circle around my left breast

and three dots—
at my sternum
and under each armpit,
cleansed with cold cotton.
"On the count of three,"
and I am tattooed
permanently
for perfect placement,
for twenty days of radiation therapy.

The needle leaves small barbaric marks—
and something like pride
unparallel
for sure
but equally as manifest in this new identity.

First Radiation Treatment

One gown goes in back,
one in front—
the starched cotton folding excessively when I sit.
I feel like baklava.

This is the secret waiting room.
This is the interior
of radiation oncology.

The woman on my right has hair.
The one on my left does not.
The first few days
we do not talk.
Our presence is too obvious.
We are redundant.

In silence, I touch an outdated copy of *People*,
hold the magazine loosely—
feign nervousness—
something to do—
like holding a drink at a party.
Or like I'm bored.
Like I do this all the time.
The cover alone
boasts of health—
of hair—
celebrity photos with long, shiny tresses.
I shield the images
from the woman on my left—
the woman with tiny, dark spikes poking
through her scalp.

I feel guilty
sitting here with hair.
I'm ashamed I don't just turn and smile.
Say hi.
Confront my vanity,

see *me* in *them*.
We're in this mess together.
And I feel stupid
hiding pictures of hair
which are suddenly too prominent,
falling out of double-page spreads,
cascading down page 43,
curling around my thumbs
and straightening my gaze.

My reach, discrete,
I tuck a tendril behind my right ear—
it's still there.
Reassurance.
Relief.
And then guilt again.

I turn pages faster
like this is hair porn—
satin over silk
bangs and highlights
blonde, brunette, ebony and auburn
foldingandslidingoverandovereachother

until my name is called.

I rise,
swish swiftly from my seat,
my inexperience
shushing the silence.

Relief walks the same path as empathy,
but I think maybe it breathes easier.

Tanning Session Twelve

A new routine:
swipe card, dressing room, starched gowns—
one in front
one in back.

She's waiting for me.
I shake one gown from my shoulders
and turn toward the mechanized table
as the gown deflates on the folding chair.

I'm a sight.
On the bottom, I wear black
Nordstrom slacks
with a belt,
and above,
my white, see-no-sun tummy
rises from the darkness—
a veneer of moon.
Fitting,
since someone painted the solar system
on the ceiling
and dimmed the lights
for "patient comfort"
like terrycloth footies at the OB-GYN.
Above my belly, my breasts—
two smaller moons—
hang loosely in suspension.
One is red
like a bad bikini burn viewed through a negative—
its sharp outlines, a rounded triangle,
sensitive to the touch.

It only takes a few minutes.
My tattoos affirm I'm aligned.
I lay still.
The machines hum and orbit around me
as isotopes emit gamma rays.

I try to concentrate on the rays
to feel warmth—
but I can't feel anything.
Weird to get sunburned
by nothing I can feel.
I wait for the machines to return
to their original positions
and study the ceiling—
imagine someone painting planets
suspended in a harness—
or just standing on a ladder—
neck crooked—
some urban Michelangelo
in a square, linoleum room off Franklin Avenue.

For a moment, I'm on my fourth grade field trip
to the planetarium,
the Museum of Nature and Science,
lounging back in the dark,
my damp ticket, a souvenir,
creased just once in my left hand.
My best friend reclines next to me,
eyeballs glossy white in her profile—
in awe.

I should have paid more attention.
I don't remember much about moons.

What else don't I remember?
What details have I discarded
carelessly
like there will always be a million more?

I sit up and swing my clothed legs to the floor
and grab my gown.
Back in the dressing room,
I slather on aloe,
feel the dent of my conspicuous scar,
clasp my bra,

button my blouse.

When I leave my planetarium,
it's sprinkling outside
and sunny.
I love this.
I want to tab this fortuity—
take in more—
catalog my gratitude.

The Receptionist at Radiation Oncology

She laughs when the glass doors whoosh me in
and tells me she fell off the bull
at the Electric Cowboy last night—
had too much fun.
I slide the caramel Frappuccino across the Formica
toward her
holding a second in my hand
and watch her eyes grow wide.
"It's 'Frappy Hour,'" I explain. "Buy One/Get One."
Cancer is an all-consuming disease.
I'm trying to live outside myself.
Her smile is wider
and she laughs again,
shows me pictures of her three kids,
sips through the green straw,
winks.
I swipe my card
and disappear into the back waiting room.
Later, on my way out,
she laughs again, knowingly.
The doors whoosh open,
my smile infecting my body,
my step, light.

Vitamin T

From the orange bottle
innocence equals pure white
but I know better.
Tamoxifen removes my estrogen
my feminine
replacing them with fatigue
and flashes of heat
warm all over
like I'm dying of embarrassment,
trapped in sheets.

I'm still me
but not quite
which is why I cried
standing in line at the pharmacy
the first time.
Five long years is a time alright.
Five long
childbearing
years,
children forbidden—
kinder verboten—
"but condoms?" I asked. "Really?"
Pills contain estrogen.
Oh.
So I waited
until after our vacation
postponing my prison—
the popping of white poison—
the first
of one thousand
eight hundred
and twenty five
more days of this
life
which

is
still
mine.

Fatigue

Never mind the ninety-minute drive.
It's the black zipper
on the suitcase
that has me paralyzed.
I haven't even started
packing.
The question of which jacket to bring
has defeated me
has me in tears, almost
which is why I'm still sitting Indian-style
on the carpet, head tilted back
against the footboard,
the roll of the mattress
like a lump on my brain.
And I'm supposed to go to the mountains to relax.

Last year
when I was eight-weeks pregnant,
remember how you steamed broccoli
and I ran to the bathroom?
The smell hasn't left me.
Then, too, I started
to pack for our weekend in Keystone,
but the minutiae of zippers
and duffel bags
and face cream
don't-forget-your-swimsuit
and the towel
and a hair tie
sunscreen,
my phone charger
left me vacant,
mouth slightly parted,
head tilted back against the hard-coiled edge
of the mattress

just like now—

waiting,
not even sure if I have energy to call you
to tell you I can't come—
won't make it.
Next time! you'll surely say,
And I'll smile,
though you can't see it on the phone,
but I know
how I am
how I'm not the same *me* that I was
before,
and I, too,
am not sure
what to make of this.

Witnessing Grace

When the time comes
will we know how to die?

My grandma never talked about her breasts.
Perhaps this was due to some element of
generational modesty—
but if you'd asked me earlier
how she passed away,
I would have replied, "Bone cancer."
Which is also true.

Her tumor, when they found it in her breast,
had metastasized.
Breasts to lymph nodes to bloodstream and beyond.
But I never heard about
her mastectomy
how she recovered
whether or not she chose to wear
a prosthesis in her bra.

When I was a little girl,
she taught me how to paint my toenails,
how to cinch a fabric purse to match my dress,
how to bake homemade bread.

Now, thirty years later,
she has shown me what it looks like
to die
gracefully.
During the last days of her life,
the breeze blew strands of beads
over the open window
by her bed,
ruffling her hair, rolled
loosely like a cinnamon bun.
She winked at me

like always,
reached for my hand,
smiled weakly,
mouthed, "I love you."

A tremendous gift.

Will I remember
how to do this
when it's my turn?

How I want to spend my time

With intention.
With resolve.
Everything, now.

Because there is not energy
for anything
extra.

And this is good.

I'm not trying to fit in *more* life.
Skip the bungee jumping—
the helicopter ride.
Last night I sat on the porch with you.
We looked at the veins
in a fallen aspen leaf, talked
about our day,
planned who'd go to Peerless tomorrow
to switch out the studded-snows.
At a soft cry from the monitor
I went upstairs in the dark to check
the crib,
returned to you,
tasted the Montepulciano you opened
and suggested who we could have over,
who we could get to know better.

Where was this welcome restriction
this social filter
a year ago
when I spent
too much time on
nothing
while trying to accomplish
everything?
What makes sense now
wasn't pertinent then.

My time is more inestimable;
more ours.

Choice
is more redeemable
when it can breathe.

Boobies

Years ago,
I helped teens volunteer
at Race for the Cure—
a worthy venture—to hold
water cups
at arm's length
and to clean up
flat, waxy cardboard—
soggy and trampled—
after the sweep of pink
passed.

How distant an event
before it applies to you.

I want to talk about my breasts
like I talk about breakfast.
I'm proud of my incision
under my armpit
with my node-negative result,
and, under my nipple,
where they removed my cancer,
my scar has slyly pursed lips
like she's holding a secret.

Hooray for bumper stickers,
T-shirts,
and bracelets I'd earlier ignored:
"I Love Boobies"
"Save the Ta-tas!"
Let there be many more to come.

Let me honor my small 34A chest.
Let me parcel my fear
with disclosed transparency.
Let me celebrate areolas.
Let me talk unabashedly,

in broad daylight,
under a cotton moon.

Plan B

My mom and I sip lattes
overlooking a Safeway parking lot.
My son, Moby-wrapped tight to me
sleeps.
We chat.
She wants me to have more children—
asks if I can—
will.
My drink is too hot.
I set it back down, a two-handed endeavor—
wipe peony lipstick from the plastic lid with my thumb.
I'm at peace with the answer
but the backs of my eyes still burn,
still need the release.

We were young when we wed.
Ten years and one miscarriage
finally gifted our little boy.
A baby is a miracle.
Bring on the clichés—
they're all true.

I always figured we would have two.
But now
this.
And five years of a drug
that will severely damage a fetus.
With risk, I could engage Plan A.
Stop the drugs. Get pregnant. Cross my fingers tight.

But when I think instead
of a child bruised by foster care,
innocent
and vulnerable,
I'm kicked in the back of the knees.
I want to answer the 2 am phone call:
"This child needs you *now*."

We'll quick make up a bed,
pull out Thomas the Train,
put on the teapot for hot chocolate,
and prepare to *love* whoever
walks in our front door
for as many minutes
hours
days
years
that we are
allowed.

I know it's not that simple,
but I *will* it to be so.

I think she understands.
This is God's way of changing my plan.
Unconventional, this possible way
of receiving and loving a second child—
unconventional,
yet limpid, untroubled—
with unforeseen clarity.

Father-in-law

Your news comes softer than mine—
I'm not sure why—
except for maybe the foreshadowing
last Tuesday
in your pale complexion
and the way your cheeks are thinning
like flat light touching snow—
evidence, they said,
of low blood count,
lack of oxygen.
Your body told you something was wrong.
Now, exactly one year after my diagnosis,
it's you
who is meeting with the oncologist.

After your appointment,
a family dinner.
We slide into the wooden booth,
stunned by blunt statements,
by spots measured in centimeters;
spleen, lungs, lymph nodes.

The hostess calls out, "Party of 6!"
hands us laminated menus—
asks what we're celebrating.

It's too soon to laugh at the irony.
Too raw to ruin the question
with an answer.

I say to myself,
We're celebrating *life*.

Literary Terms

We're studying short stories—
their elements,
intended effects,
their structure.
Literature is full of life
and death and second chances,
love and fate
and change.
Antagonists, asides,
and what I'm really getting to:
the *climax* of the story.

These freshmen rattle off terms
like they understand.
"The climax is the *most exciting* part of the story,"
they announce
and settle into their desks,
ready for resolution.

And here's where I stop them.
"The *most exciting* part?" I muse.
"Yeah."
They are ready to move on,
satisfied with quick assessment.

I know what they're thinking:
Exciting implies gore and carnage,
debilitating injuries,
heart-wrenching break-ups.
Like Romeo in Act III.
In a rage because Tybalt has killed his best friend,
Romeo retaliates,
thrusts his sword through Tybalt's gut,
sticky now,
warm and crimson.
If Romeo had been a vampire,
Shakespeare would have nailed it.

But "exciting" has nothing to do with climax.
We often miss the point.
We think we understand.
But we move
too fast
think too fast
act too fast
and die
too
fast.

"The definition of climax is not *the-most-exciting-part*,
it's the *turning point*."

This changes everything.
There is no restoring of innocence.
Nothing can be the same.
The point of no return.
The story
must *change*.

Beautiful, isn't it?

My cancer, too.
A blessing to my story.
A richness.
My *turning point*
which can still mean anything.

At present
I feel chronologically at large
with loose narrative structure.

A reward, this
irresolution.

Anthem of Hope

My cancer is on loan,
its effects doled out to me in tiny pleated paper cups—
its origin still a mystery.
It has made its mark—
affected change—
proved its power.

So now, I vow not
to sit, ankles crossed,
stare, fixed;
hardened.
Let's talk instead about fluidity:
stratus clouds
and flooding rivers that have autonomy
to run free,
change maps.
Let's talk about interconnectedness;
belonging.
I will not live for myself
and if I think for one moment
that I'm in control,
you'd better challenge me with *Of what?*

I must fashion my foundation on granite and shale, both.
From what is certain
and from what crumbles
under the rubber sole of my boot.
The sickness of an easy life
is not curable
save with hardship.

My prayers are more fervent now,
dogged like spring leaves,
warm and sticky with a baited question.

But see the white flag raised high?
How it ripples under the wind's derision?

It stands tall
and forfeits
control.

Solder together
the fragments,
minutes,
hours,
days of my fear,
and see how this sum equals hope—
how uncertainty ushers vitality—

how acceptance heals.

Cancer's Timeline

Sunday, Feb. 26, 2012	Discovered lump in breast
Tuesday, Feb. 28	Appointment with OB-GYN to check lump and remove IUD
Wednesday, Feb. 29	First mammogram and ultrasound
Friday, Mar. 2	Biopsy and second post-biopsy mammogram
Wednesday, Mar. 7	Received "the phone call"— carcinoma present
Friday, Mar. 9	(All day appointments) MRI, chest x-ray, and consultations with the surgeon, oncologist, and nurse
Wednesday, Mar. 14	Ultrasound to confirm MRI. Two more tumors in question
Thursday, Mar. 15	MRI biopsy on second suspected lump on same side and third post-biopsy mammogram
Friday, Mar. 23	Surgery: lumpectomy and sentinel node biopsy
Friday, Apr. 6	Follow-up appointment with surgeon to discuss pathology report
Monday, Apr. 9	Consultation with oncologist to discuss treatment options: chemotherapy, radiation, and Tamoxifen

Tuesday, Apr. 10	Oncologist calls with low Oncotype score which potentially changes plans for treatment
Tuesday, Apr. 17	Consultation with radiation oncologist
Thursday, Apr. 19	First radiation set-up and tattoos applied
Monday, Apr. 23	Blood test and consultation with the genetic counseling department
Tuesday, Apr. 24	Call from oncologist with results from the "tumor board" who reviewed my case: all doctors present cannot agree whether chemotherapy would be beneficial or detrimental for me
Friday, May 5	Second radiation set-up and x-rays
Monday, May 7	Consultation with the genetic counseling department: test results show I tested negative for both the BRCA 1 and 2 genes
	Decision made *not* to have a mastectomy and to continue solely with radiation, *not* chemotherapy
Monday, May 7	Fourth mammogram for post-surgery base pictures
Tuesday, May 8	Start of radiation treatments: everyday for twenty days at 4:00 pm.

Wednesday, May 9   2nd radiation treatment

Thursday, May 10   3rd radiation treatment

Friday, May 11   4th radiation treatment

Monday, May 14   5th radiation treatment

Tuesday, May 15   6th radiation treatment

Wednesday, May 16   7th radiation treatment

Thursday, May 17   8th radiation treatment

Friday, May 18   9th radiation treatment

Monday, May 21   10th radiation treatment

Tuesday, May 22   11th radiation treatment

Wednesday, May 23   12th radiation treatment

Thursday, May 24   13th radiation treatment

Friday, May 25   14th radiation treatment

Tuesday, May 29   15th radiation treatment

Wednesday, May 30   16th radiation treatment

Thursday, May 31   17th radiation treatment

Friday, Jun. 1   18th radiation treatment

Monday, Jun. 4   19th radiation treatment and our
                      12th wedding anniversary

Tuesday, Jun. 5   20th radiation treatment

Tuesday, Jul. 3   Consultation with oncologist to discuss hormone treatment and future check-ups

Afterword

"Remission" is a beautiful word with a confusing connotation. Six months after surgery, radiation, and the start of Tamoxifen, I scheduled an MRI as a final check—to ensure that, indeed, the cancer was no longer active in my body.

The MRI itself was cake (I had already had three)—but its looming appointment had made me nauseous, and after the MRI, I had to wait two more weeks for the results. And they wouldn't just call me with the results—I had to schedule another appointment. I feared more than anything that their reasoning for this was because often a patient must receive bad news—or the possibility of "a question," and maybe receiving bad news *in person* is better. I had just started teaching again for the new school year, and I couldn't fathom the possible need for "more testing."

So my clean result, then, was a welcome relief, and in a weird way, a shock. It almost didn't seem possible that all of my fears over the past six months could be erased with the words of my radiation-oncologist: "Technically, you can say that you're now in remission." I didn't know what remission *technically* meant, but it sounded good. It sounded *done*. I looked it up when I got home. It loosely means that the signs of cancer have completely disappeared (although that sneaky definition won't come clean about whether this is a temporary or a permanent state). Regardless, "remission" was all I could ask for and hope for.

While the congratulatory-remission-concept is certainly something to be celebrated, it comes with another side which I'll break down into three parts:

Remission, Part I: Released

I name this part with both fondness and irony. I remember back when I delivered my little boy. Having a baby is, perhaps, an odd, but appropriate analogy for Part I. For nine months of pregnancy, fear, excitement, and anxiety were braided together, and everything in my life funneled into one, tiny due date—the end all of end-alls—at which point the baby came. I was sore, still bleeding, and could hardly walk; I was blurry eyed, sleep-deprived, and my nipples were starting to chap from trying to breast-feed. The sleeper I brought to take him home in was too big, and all I wanted was a shower. Ironically, it was at this moment when I barely had it together that they asked me to sign my "release" papers. Ha. I was done. Or, more appropriately, *they* were done with *me*. I'd been released. And as any mom knows, *that* was when real motherhood began. The trials (and the joys) were just beginning. My husband and I were on our own. The medical world was done with us.

I felt this same way during that appointment when I heard I was in "remission." I wasn't really *done*—but the medical world was done with me. "Schedule a mammogram once per year, and continue regular check-ups with your OB-GYN"—and, void of suspicious activity, these new doctors of mine were fading photographs in my memory.

Remission, Part II: Doing Dishes

Of all the "chores," I like "dishes" best. Maybe because of the warm water—because I'm always cold. I like the dull noise of a running faucet. It soothes me. And doing dishes affirms normalcy. Ahh. Finally. "Dishes" is a sigh of relief.

It's taken awhile for these normal bits of life to come back. Not that I didn't do dishes for six months—somehow I must have—but it certainly didn't occur in any normal sense. Our house was perpetually disorganized. Daily living was too overwhelming in the aura of our greater concerns. Sometimes my husband just ran to Chipotle for take-out so we wouldn't have to make dinner or clean up.

But we were so numb. It was as if, after eating, we couldn't figure out what to do with the trash.

It feels so good to do dishes again…and pay the bills and take the car to the car wash and sweep dust from the hardwood floors after leaving the windows open for too many breezy, summer nights.

At this stage, the cliché "Live life to the fullest" means, for me, "Revel in mediocrity." What do I mean? The completion of mundane, daily tasks is, unexpectedly, a privilege. I'm here. I'm still alive. I *get* to run these errands, go to the bank. I *get* to build a train track around the coffee table. I *get* to sweep the porch and sit next to my husband after my son goes to bed. I love the commonplace.

I remember one specific evening sitting in traffic heading north into Boulder, the orange construction cones stretching out like buoys. The sun was setting behind the mountains on my left, and the haze over the city on my right blurred the outlines of commerce. The earth felt overexposed. And I got to participate. I was still in the game. Six months earlier, I would have been exasperated by my elongated commute. That day, I understood that I still got to play. I relaxed. Enjoyed the scenery. Turned off the engine. Rolled down the windows. Checked over my right shoulder at my son, asleep in his car seat, head nodding sideways. Mundane life. Normal life. Beautiful life.

Remission, Part III: Tempering the beast

As of this writing, I have three years left of taking Tamoxifen to reduce my risk of getting cancer again. After those three years are up, I still don't think I'll ever feel free of fear. Although my body is done with treatments, my mind hasn't yet chosen to let go.

The fear of recurrence is a spirited beast. It heightens my anxiety and keeps me awake at night. I want to say that the fear of recurrence "haunts" me. Because it does. I think about the word "cancer" every day. (The doctors forgot to *release* me from its connotations and the burden of its six letters.) I've been given the "all-clear," but all I can think about is whether I'll be able to teach my son to ride his bike, and, if the cancer comes back and I die, whether he'll remember how I'd make up songs about trains and strum them on the guitar while he danced in circles around me on the carpet.

Unfortunately, my father-in-law passed away from cancer recently, too, just four months after his diagnosis. We miss him dearly. Though we're consoled that he's home in heaven, his loss reminds me of how lucky I am that I caught my cancer so early.

I'll never understand why I got breast cancer at such a young age (or even at all)—I'm just a "normal" woman. But I think I'm a better person now because of it. And I've learned a few things.

To start, I've learned not to read cancer-related websites (especially not before I go to bed) because they all say I'm surely going to die. I've learned not to read too many books. Health and medicine-related topics seem to evolve too frequently, and the contrasting opinions are too overwhelming to me. I've learned that lists of symptoms do not apply to everyone—that diseases try to box people in—but that our bodies react individually to every aspect of life, including cancer. For example, fatigue is the symptom that I struggle with most on a daily basis, but it's listed under the "rare" symptoms of Tamoxifen. And some of the other common symptoms skirted by me.

I've also learned that I can't plan my life. I'm a "planner" by nature—it's what I love most about my career. Cancer is a rude disease and takes no note of another's so-called plans. Though having another child is certainly a possibility, my husband and I probably won't risk getting pregnant again. Our plans have changed, and this is ok. And I've learned to put more trust in God, the only one who understands *any* plan for my life or for the lives of those with whom I come into contact.

In light of my decreased energy and desire to ensure that what I *do* spend time on *counts*, I've learned to ask the question, *Will my life be better for this?* Yesterday, I chose to say "no" to making a second trip to Home Depot to select complimentary paint samples, and "no" to running to the grocery store last minute before dinner (I changed the menu, and since we already had milk and eggs at home, I made French toast for dinner instead). And I say "yes" to things that will enrich my life or someone else's life: helping my parents tile their new bathroom, reading bedtime stories to my son, being invited to dinner. I need to ask myself more frequently, *How can I get the rest I need for myself,* and *Who, today, can I deliberately choose to show love?* A few days ago, I ordered a double-tall latte at Starbucks with my friend, and we talked about *her*. Not me. Not cancer. It was wonderful.

I'm sensitive to my husband's journey with my breast cancer, as well. It's not over for him, either. He was and is my rock. But he has the same fears. And he has to adjust to a somewhat-different, less-energetic *me*. Together we understand the divergence from our precancer life, and we've teamed up to love the life we have with each other. What that means is different every day.

Because getting cancer seems to be somewhat random (like getting in a car accident—its effects equally as deadly, equally as common), ultimately, the cancer-beast is mollified solely by my attitude. My response to cancer, to my fatigue, to my fear, and to those I love *matters*. Everything about who I am is wrapped in this response. Cancer cannot be controlled, so I pray that I respond well, live well, and love well, no matter what the future holds.

ACKNOWLEDGMENTS

Without my loving husband, Orrin, standing next to me through every element of my breast-cancer diagnosis, the seeds of this memoir would surely have blown away.

Heartfelt gratitude also to Julie Pouliot, Corrie Knapp, and Dave Cohara for reading and editing poem after poem through various stages of completion. Without their encouragement and methodical, critical feedback, this would not have been possible.

And to my parents, Tom and Marti Pouliot, for their never-ending love and support in all my endeavors.

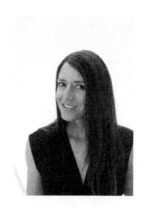

ABOUT THE AUTHOR

Amy Burns holds a master's degree in humanities and teaches English at the high school level. Her cancer is in remission. She lives in Golden, Colorado with her husband and three year-old son.

Please email breastcancerat35@gmail.com to share responses and personal experiences. Select responses may be included in a future edition. Thank you!

CPSIA information can be obtained at www.ICGtesting.com
Printed in the USA
LVOW04s1009260415

436147LV00020B/1242/P